Zebras of Hope

Table of Contents

Zebras of Hope

Introduction

Shortly after my diagnosis of Ehlers-Danlos syndrome (EDS), I came to realize that there were no books dedicated to coping with the pain and suffering that comes with the diagnosis. Being diagnosed with an incurable disease is a frightening experience, and deserves to be recognized as such. We zebras need to know that we are not alone; we need sources for sharing coping strategies, difficulties, and successes.

Some of you reading this may not know why I am using the term zebra to describe those afflicted with Ehlers-Danlos syndrome. A medical zebra is someone with a rare diagnosis. In medical school doctors are taught that when they hear hoof beats they should think horses not zebras. Therefore many doctors will miss a rare diagnosis because they only concentrate on the obvious.

I was diagnosed with EDS several years ago. My initial reaction to being diagnosed with Ehlers-Danlos syndrome was relief. I was relieved that there was a name to go along with all the symptoms I had been suffering with for years. Soon thereafter, however, I was overcome with grief for the life I knew I would not be able to live the way I had planned. Hiking backcountry trails and working with wild black bears would be out of the question. I would have to create new life plans and goals. Learning to accept my limitations was the hardest part of the diagnosis.

As I write this I am sitting in bed and living on disability insurance, something I never thought would happen to me. I was the girl who went to the gym five days a week, tried to eat right, and followed all the latest nutritional advice. I read Shape magazine to keep up on all the current health trends. Yet when EDS started to break down my body, there was no stopping it with exercise or nutrition. Typing and using a mouse became too difficult for me to do regularly. I'm typing this book using DragonDictate. I am learning new ways to take my life back and become independent again.

I hope to use this book as a way to show zebras who have been newly diagnosed that there is hope for a fulfilling life and room for joy.

Part I

Chapter 1

What is Ehlers-Danlos syndrome?

This book is not about the medical aspects of Ehlers-Danlos syndrome (EDS); it is about living with Ehlers-Danlos syndrome. Yet, it is important for me to give a brief overview of EDS and the different subtypes. I am not a medical professional, and the information presented here was obtained through research and my personal knowledge gained through living with EDS and communicating with other EDS patients and families.

Ehlers-Danlos was first described by Dr. Job Janszoon van Meek'ren in 1682, and later described by Drs. Edvard Ehlers and Henri-Alexandre Danlos in 1901 and 1908, Ehlers-Danlos syndrome is a disease caused by a mutation of the genes[1]. This mutation results in faulty collagen, the basic supporting protein in connective tissue. Collagen is a fibrous protein which provides strength and elasticity to the bones, ligaments, tendons, skin, organ linings, and blood vessel walls, all of which are connective tissue and can be affected by this genetic disease.[6] There are several different defects known which can cause Ehlers-Danlos syndrome. Prior to 1997, Ehlers-Danlos syndrome was broken down into eleven types which were given corresponding Roman numerals. The classification system was revised during a meeting in Villefranche, France by experts: Peter Beighton, Anne De Paepe, Beat Steinmann, Petros Tsipouras, and Richard J. Wenstrup in 1997, creating a simpler classification system based on symptoms. Under the new system, there are six major subtypes of Ehlers-Danlos syndrome. These subtypes run true to a family, meaning that if I have classical type, I could not pass on vascular type to my children.[2]

The subtypes of Ehlers-Danlos syndrome are: hypermobility (formerly type III), classical (formerly types I and II), vascular (formerly type IV), kyphoscoliosis (formerly type VI), arthrochalasia (formerly type VIIB), and dermatosparaxis (formerly type VIIC).[2] There are other even rarer forms of the disease, some of which are only known to exist in single families, but I will not go into any of those here.

Hypermobile type involves the hypermobility of both large and small joints. There may be some skin involvement; including hyperextensible skin and/or smooth/velvety skin, as well as easy bruising. At the present time, there is no genetic testing available for the hypermobile type. Therefore, diagnosis must be made through clinical criteria, including the Beighton Scale (a diagnostic tool for measuring joint hypermobility) and skin involvement. Some doctors are reluctant to give an EDS diagnosis to a patient with hypermobile type, and prefer to diagnose them with Generalized Joint Hypermobility Syndrome, Joint Hypermobility Syndrome, or Benign Joint Hypermobility Syndrome. The biggest problem patients seem to have with the latter diagnosis is that it minimizes their disease by calling it "benign" and therefore this diagnosis is no longer being used according to some experts, however, I was diagnosed with it before receiving the corrected diagnosis of classical type EDS, so it is still being used by some geneticists. A study conducted in 2009 found that there is no clinical distinction between the hypermobile type of EDS[3] and the Hypermobility Syndromes mentioned above.

Classical type also involves both the skin and the joints, but with the added likelihood of extensive scarring, organ prolapses, and hernias in children. COL5A1, COL5A2, and COL1A1 are the genes that have been identified in classical EDS[4]. Unfortunately, skin biopsies are not sensitive enough to identify all cases, although they may be helpful to confirm a diagnosis[1].

Vascular type may have some hypermobility of the small joints, skin involvement including very poor wound healing, thin translucent skin, extensive bruising, characteristic facial appearance, and a shortened life expectancy. The median age of death for a patient with vascular EDS is 48 years. These deaths are most often caused by ruptured arteries or ruptured organs.[5] COL3A1 is the gene responsible for vascular EDS[4], and a skin biopsy can be used to identify more than 95% of individuals affected with EDS vascular type[1].

Kyphoscoliosis type involves scoliosis at birth that worsens with age, generalized joint laxity, severe muscle hypotonia at birth, osteopenia[4], fragile skin and eyes, possible blood vessel involvement, and a possible decrease in bone mass[1]. PLOD1 is the gene responsible for the kyphoscoliosis type of EDS[4], and it can be found through laboratory testing of the urine[1].

Arthrochalasia type involves congenital bilateral hip dislocations (both hips are dislocating at birth), severe generalized hypermobility, highly stretchable skin that bruises easily, and scarring[4]. The genes responsible for arthrochalasia type are COL1A1 and COL1A2[4]. A skin biopsy and direct DNA testing are available for diagnosis of arthrochalasia type.

Dermatosparaxis type is marked by skin fragility without excessive scarring, sagging and/or soft skin, easy bruising, large hernias, and premature rupture of fetal membranes[4]. ADAMTS2 is the gene responsible for dermatosparaxis type[4]. Skin biopsies are available for diagnosis[1].

There is much crossover among types of EDS. Someone afflicted with vascular type may have crossover characteristics of hypermobile type, just as a person with hypermobile type may exhibit signs of classical type. There may be a great deal of symptom discrepancy even among members of the same family. Therefore, typing will remain difficult until all responsible genes have been identified.

Hypermobile, classical, vascular, and arthrochalasia types are autosomal dominant[1]. This means that each child of someone with EDS has a 50% chance of being born with the disease.[6] If a parent with EDS has more than one child, each additional child has that same 50% chance of being born with the disease. Kyphoscoliosis and dermatosparaxis are autosomal recessive[4].

It is believed that one in 5,000 people have the most common form of Ehlers-Danlos syndrome, hypermobility type, two to five in 100,000 people have classical type, one in 100,000 to 250,000 have vascular Ehlers-Danlos syndrome, and all other types of Ehlers-Danlos syndrome are rarer still[4].

Chapter 2

Symptoms

Chronic pain is a daily symptom for most people with Ehlers-Danlos syndrome. Imaging studies such as x-rays and MRIs often show no abnormalities. This can be very frustrating for both doctors and patients, as they know that something is wrong but have difficulty identifying the exact cause of the pain. Brad T. Tinkle, M.D., Ph.D., a clinical geneticist with Advocate Medical Group - Park Ridge in Park Ridge, Illinois, who specializes in connective tissue diseases and has written two books about Ehlers-Danlos syndrome hypermobility type says "loose joints can cause stress/strain on the surrounding ligaments and tendons which may cause pain. This is often worse when bones move out of their joints. Muscle pain is also part of the overall pain due to the overuse. Eventually, chronic pain may cause nerve sensation and amplification of the pain." (B. Tinkle, personal communication, August 2, 2012).

It has been suggested to many of us who suffer with Ehlers-Danlos syndrome (EDSers) by our doctors that our extreme pain may be due to a secondary condition of fibromyalgia, which causes a higher degree of pain perception. Studies have suggested that there may be abnormalities in the central nervous system such as the levels of chemicals in the cerebrospinal fluid which transmits pain signals to and from the brain[7]. There is some controversy within the EDS community over whether fibromyalgia is the cause of the increased pain or pain perception among EDS patients. Some believe that fibromyalgia is a misdiagnosis in most EDS patients, and that their symptoms are more likely to be caused solely by their EDS. Others suggest that fibromyalgia is simply more common in the EDS community. There is quite a bit of overlap in symptoms in both disorders, including: widespread pain, muscle soreness, fatigue, anxiety, depression, migraines, and sleep disturbance. Treatments for EDS and fibromyalgia can also be similar, and include finding ways to treat the individual symptoms, such as improving sleep hygiene, reducing stress, low-impact physical therapy, and finding medications to ease pain.

Whatever its cause, chronic pain can take a severe toll on our physical and mental health. Finding ways to deal with chronic pain takes time, patience, and perseverance. For most, it will take a combination of therapies to lessen the effects of chronic pain, such as: medication, heat therapy, massage, physical and occupational therapy, as well as relaxation and stress management techniques.

In some cases, physicians believe patients are exaggerating their pain, and may even label them as displaying "drug seeking behavior." Other times physicians will refer the patient for mental health evaluation, as if the pain is "all in their head." Some EDSers have been labeled as malingerers and hypochondriacs prior to getting an EDS diagnosis. Because most tests, such as MRIs and x-rays come up normal, it can be difficult to diagnose EDS, and, therefore, doctors may mistake the wide-array of symptoms and complaints of an EDS patient for malingering. If you suspect you or a loved one has EDS, getting to a geneticist trained in identifying EDS is an essential first step in receiving proper diagnosis and treatment. These specialists are usually booked months in advance, but after years of suffering with pain and frustration, waiting those months will be well worth the expert opinion.

Chronic hand pain makes typing difficult and can lead to loss of work. Large companies are usually willing to make accommodations for disabilities in accordance with the law, at least in the U.S. But even with accommodations work is not always possible. Because the pain that an EDSer feels will often change depending on the joint being used, changing careers may not solve the problem either. For example, if you spend time on your feet while working a cash register or waiting tables, your toes, knees, and hips may become your primary problem, with subluxations and dislocations of those joints causing pain in the lower extremities. Yet, if you are using your hands and arms while typing, washing dishes, or folding laundry, you may have dislocations and subluxations of those joints, thus causing you to feel the pain in your shoulders, elbows, hands, wrists, and fingers. The joints that you use the most often are likely to be the ones that cause you the most significant pain.

As mentioned above, joint instability is one of the causes of chronic pain in EDS. Frequent subluxations and dislocations of both small and large joints, not only bring about intense sharp pain, but also present other challenges. Seemingly simple things, such as: getting out of bed, dressing, brushing hair, pouring a cup of coffee, and lifting a bowl to give pets water, can result in joints popping out of place. Braces may help keep joints in place, and enable you to accomplish some of these small activities. However, bracing is not always practical. Bracing the hip joint is not practical, and because of that, many will have problems with their hips subluxing frequently, even from small activities like putting on a pair of pants or walking to the bathroom. Shoulder bracing is sometimes ineffective, and the shoulder may still pop out with the brace on, which means having to limit activities involving the shoulder. Limiting activities can then result in loss of muscle tone, which then leads to more frequent subluxations and dislocations, so it is quite a challenge to determine the best course of action, and must be decided on an individual basis.

In addition to joint issues and chronic pain, EDSers must cope with unusual skin problems. Small mishaps can result in severe bruising, which may cause embarrassment, or far worse, may even lead to child-abuse accusations. I once bumped the corner of my eye while on a cruise vacation and spent the rest of the cruise enduring stares from people who thought my husband had punched me. At the time, the experience was mortifying, though time passing has left me with an amusing story to share with friends. For parents unfairly accused of child-abuse, there is no amusement to speak of. Normal play can result in the severe bruising and scarring, which may cause teachers and coaches to assume the worst, and report suspected child abuse to authorities. Having a diagnosis, along with informative literature to pass along to teachers, camp counselors, babysitters, and church leaders can help diffuse some of those situations.

Another common symptom is of Ehlers-Danlos Syndrome is fatigue. This is not just normal tiredness, but rather a severe loss of energy. A person experiencing fatigue may have difficulty accomplishing simple tasks, and always feel run-down, overwhelmed, and exhausted.

Many EDSers also suffer from bowel disorders, such as irritable bowel syndrome (IBS) and constipation. Some EDSers have episodes of severe spasms and diarrhea. However, on the other end of the spectrum, those on medications for chronic pain may suffer from chronic constipation. Prolapse of the rectum is also possible, and will most often require surgery to correct. The prolapse is often precipitated by constipation; the excessive straining combined with the already lax connective tissue results in a prolapse. Bowel issues are an uncomfortable topic that many of us don't even want to bring up with our doctors, but they can be serious, so they need to be addressed.

Dental problems may also be significant among the EDS population, including: hypermobility of the temporomandibular joint, overcrowding, excessive bleeding during dental procedures, problems with oral sutures not holding, tooth fragility, and premature loss of teeth due to early onset periodontitis[8]. EDS patients may also absorb numbing medications, such as Novocain rapidly, and, consequently, the medication may wear off during procedures, which may result in EDSers choosing to avoid the dentist due to a fear of the pain the procedures might cause.

Commonly, EDSers will suffer from secondary conditions such as an autonomic disorder, the most frequent among EDSers being Postural Orthostatic Tachycardia Syndrome (POTS). Autonomic dysfunction can include problems such as low blood pressure, light-headedness, fatigue, and syncope. Like EDS itself, the symptoms can range from somewhat mild to quite severe, depending on the individual patient. Most POTS patients need to be followed by a cardiologist and must take daily medications to control their POTS symptoms. It can take months or even years before the doctors find the right combination of medications to ease POTS symptoms.

Early onset osteoarthritis and osteoporosis are also more common to the EDS population.

Much of the frustration of patients with EDS stems from the fact that for many of us, EDS is an invisible illness, which means that others cannot see our medical condition through its physical manifestations. Some of us use a cane or wheel chair, which helps to identify us as having a physical problem, but most EDSers look just like the rest of the population. Invisible illnesses have their own set of challenges. When someone has a visible disease, they are more likely to receive kind words and assistance from others. When your disease is invisible, others cannot see it, and therefore do not offer the same kind considerations that they offer to those with visible illnesses. For example, when walking across a parking lot, cars will get more impatient when someone without a cane or wheelchair moves rather slowly. Also, when parking in handicap spots, people with invisible illnesses will often be looked at strangely or even yelled at by others who cannot see their handicap. Therefore, living with an invisible illness can be a serious challenge indeed.

Chapter 3

Long Road to Diagnosis

When dealing with a rare disease, the search for diagnosis can be long and arduous. The average time from bringing symptoms to a doctor's attention to receiving a diagnosis for a rare disease is more than seven years according to a study done by Shire[9]. The hypermobile type of EDS really is not all that rare, with one in five thousand being thought to have it. However, the other types of EDS are very rare, and are even less easily diagnosed than the hypermobile type.

One of the reasons for the difficulty in diagnosing EDS is that there can be a wide range of symptoms and severity even within the same family. Two children from the same family may experience varying degrees of disability. One may have mild hand and arm pain. The other may have disabling knee and hip problems. It can be difficult for doctors to connect those problems, especially if they do not have both family members as patients. What typically happens is that one person in a family finally gets a diagnosis, finds out that it is a genetic disease, and reads up on the possible symptoms, and that is how they find out that other family members have symptoms of the disease.

Another reason for the difficulty in diagnosing EDS is that a patient may report to the doctor with symptoms that seem completely unrelated, so the doctor assumes that the patient has two or three differing problems, as opposed to one all encompassing problem. An example of this would be a young woman reporting with a prolapsed uterus, hand pain, and severe headaches. In most cases, a patient with those types of varied symptoms does have three different problems, but with EDS they are all connected because they are all resulting from the missing collagen in the connective tissue.

So, although it would be easy to become angry at the multitude of doctors we have been referred to prior to receiving a diagnosis, and to get angry about the misdiagnoses we receive prior to receiving the correct diagnosis, it is counter-productive to allow ourselves to wallow in the anger and frustration. We can better serve ourselves by trying to understand the frustration of the various specialists we have seen, and how many of them have honestly wanted to help us, and simply did not have enough information or training in the field of connective tissue diseases to understand what our symptoms indicated. Of course, having said that, it is still inexcusable behavior for a physician to berate a patient with EDS and accuse them of drug seeking behavior when they speak of their pain levels. Physicians have a responsibility to treat patients with respect and to seek real answers, not to just throw a generic diagnosis at us and hope we go away. A couple of frequent misdiagnoses of EDS patients are fibromyalgia and chronic pain syndrome, while these can be sister diseases, which are caused by EDS, they are not the "cause" of our problems, so we have to be careful accepting such labels, being sure to advocate for ourselves until we are correctly diagnosed.

When first receiving an EDS diagnosis, the initial feeling is often relief. We are so glad to finally have a name to go with the symptoms. Physicians can no longer tell us that we are hypochondriacs or that our pain is caused by depression, or some other mental diagnosis. The relief is very real, and may last a few days to a few months depending on the person. Unfortunately, the initial excitement and elation at receiving a diagnosis does not usually last. Many of us will mourn the loss of our dreams for our lives. When you realize that there is no cure to your disease, and that you will never recover from it, it can be devastating. We need to take the time to express our feelings, without wallowing in them. It can be easy to get lost in depression, but there is a way out. To get out of depression and stay out of that depression, we need to learn to accept our diagnosis and our limitations, and learn to plan our lives around those limitations. I am not suggesting it is easy. I am suggesting that it is an absolute necessity. Everyone has a different way of learning to cope. I lean on the Lord, because He will never let me down, and I encourage everyone to do the same. However, I recognize that some people will choose to lean entirely on friends and family, and some will choose to get psychiatric help. God is the only stable force that I know I can rely on, so that is the path I choose. As long as I am willing, He will allow me to lean on Him. His love gets me through every day, and gives me the strength to be positive most of the time.

Part II

Zebras before you (the personal stories from other EDSers)

This section contains the personal stories, documenting the challenges ad successes of patients diagnosed with Ehlers-Danlos Syndrome. In collecting and editing these stories, I have learned that these patients are resilient and strong, and have amazing character. Living through pain and frustration can make us stronger, if we choose to let it, and these patients chose to make the most of life with Ehlers-Danlos Syndrome, and live their lives to the fullest. I will start this section by sharing my own personal story from struggling to find a diagnosis to learning to live my life again.

My EDS Story (Classical Type)

My name is Ellen Kelleher, I am a 41 year old mother of one. I have a loving husband, an old dog, two sheep, three goats, and thirteen chickens. I also have a supportive extended family, but Ehlers-Danlos Syndrome has dramatically changed my life.

As I began my adult life, I started having frequent joint, bone, and nerve pain. I worked in an office environment doing legal work and administrative tasks, as well as technical support. These jobs all involved extensive keyboard and mouse use, which caused extreme pain in my arms, wrists, hands, and fingers. I mistakenly believed that I had Carpal Tunnel Syndrome.

My doctor suggested I have an EMG to test for nerve damage, but I put this off for more than five years. When I finally had the EMG, it was negative, so I had to have another one done, which was also negative. They then ordered numerous other tests, which were also all negative. Eventually, I was referred to a rheumatologist who saw me for about 3 minutes before he decided I had Ehlers-Danlos Syndrome (hypermobile type).

From there, I went to a geneticist to confirm. He suggested it wasn't Ehlers-Danlos Syndrome, that it was Benign Familial Hypermobility Syndrome. I wasn't sure what to make of that diagnosis, as there was very little available online about that disease. About a year later, I did a search on Amazon for a book on Hypermobility Syndrome. That is how I first found Dr. Brad Tinkle's book *Issues and Management of Joint Hypermobility: A Guide for the Ehlers-Danlos Syndrome Hypermobility Type and the Hypermobility Syndrome*. In reading this book, I learned that there was a school of thought in the medical community that perhaps the Hyermobility Syndrome and EDS Hypermobile type were the same disease. Since that time, Dr. Tinkle worked with other leading geneticists to prepare an extensive research paper on that subject.

In reading Dr. Tinkle's book, I found that it explained everything I had experienced, from the pain in all of my joints to my digestive problems, and more. I finally felt understood, and it was a huge relief. Dr. Tinkle now has another book out called *Joint Hypermobility Handbook- A Guide for the Issues & Management of Ehlers-Danlos*

Syndrome Hypermobility Type and the Hypermobility Syndrome. It covers all the same symptoms as the first book, but goes further, by adding more detailed information on coping strategies and treatment options.

After reading Dr. Tinkle's first book, I decided I needed a second opinion from a geneticist, so I sought out the best of the best. I was torn between going to Cincinatti, Ohio to see Brad Tinkle, M.D. and going to Baltimore, Maryland to see Clair A. Francomano, M.D. I chose to see Dr. Francomano because she was closer to home. She is truly a one of a kind doctor. After spending a great deal of time with me, going over family history and symptoms, as well as performing a physical exam, she changed my diagnosis to Ehlers-Danlos Classical type. She explained that because I had experienced bladder and pelvic organ prolapse, a miscarriage, had a high palate, soft auricles, problems with my teeth, and somewhat stretchy skin, that I was a better fit in the classical type, even though my Beighton score was 9 out of 9. (The Beighton score is a standardized test used to determine the extent of an individual's hypermobility.) My brother, Richard, went with me to that appointment, and he also fit well into the classical category.

My mother, my little sister, and my son, have all shown signs of EDS as well. My son has wide scarring on his legs, and has already begun dislocating his knee and his hip. My little sister has had problems with ovarian cysts, and has quite a bit of hypermobility. My mother has many of the same symptoms I do.

18

My brother, Richard, is ten years my junior. He has been having serious medical problems since he was a teenager. He had extreme debilitating chest pain, which kept him from being able to work or attend school at times. He eventually had to grow accustomed to the pain, as the doctors were not able to diagnose the cause of his pain. As he has aged, he has developed even more serious problems including a total loss of cartilage in his spine, and he developed a "hump." He has problems with his hips and had to have a labral tear repaired. The repair involved painful surgery with a very long recovery, during which he experienced an even greater degree of pain, as well as hip dislocations from simple everyday things, such as sitting in a chair! He is considering a total hip replacement in the future.

My shoulder used to pop in and out several times a day, so I had shoulder stabilization surgery to correct it. At first, I visited a local surgeon who refused to treat me because of my Ehlers-Danlos Syndrome and the possible complications.

Eventually, I found a surgeon who was willing to treat me. He performed an open surgical repair to correct instability in my left shoulder done. The recovery was very difficult and painful, and the surgery seemed to be successful for about six months before it began to fail. Now the joint is again subluxing regularly, but I still think it is better than prior to the surgery. I also underwent open surgery to repair my bladder prolapse and pelvic prolapse. The surgery for that was also a success. I had an ablation to relieve heavy bleeding and address low iron anemia and increased POTS symptoms.

More seriously, however, Richard and I both had to undergo three major spinal surgeries with neurosurgeon, Fraser Henderson, M.D. Dr. Henderson performed surgery to correct a basilar invagination and cranio-cervical instability. A few years before that, he de-tethered both of our spinal cords, and he did surgery to correct problems with our cervical spines as well. Richard needed to have one entire vertebrae removed and replaced. I had veterbrae fused together at C4/C5. After the surgery, both of us had problems with blood clots from the IV... my clots resolved on their own, but Richard had to have another surgery to have his removed. I continue to have numbness on the right side of my head following the last surgery. I am grateful for a surgeon like Dr. Henderson, who loves the Lord. My faith in Dr. Henderson's abilities was greatly increased by my knowledge that God is with him as he works.

I see many different doctors to monitor my various symptoms: neurologist, neurosurgeon, cardiologist, rheumatologist, pulmonologist, geneticist, urogynecologist, internist, endocrinologist, physiatrist, and orthopedist. It seems every doctor I see refers me to at least one additional specialist, and sometimes orders several new tests, treatments, or therapies too. It is a busy life, and had caused me to miss quite a bit of work before I finally went out on disability.

In addition to my Ehlers-Danlos Syndrome, I have several other related conditions, including:

Postural Orthostatic Tachycardia Syndrome (POTS), osteoarthritis, scoliosis, asthma, tethered-cord syndrome (now de-tethered), cranio-cervical instability and basilar invagination (surgically stabilized), gastroparesis, hypomotility, irritable bowel syndrome, suspected Mast Cell Activation Disorder (MCAD) and degenerative disc disease. All of these are believed to be more common in Ehlers-Danlos patients due to the collagen defect which causes EDS. I used to take many different medications to treat my symptoms, but due to severe digestive issues, I now only take what I need the most, medications for my digestive system and medications to stabilize my heart rate and blood pressure. I have not found a medication which will alleviate my pain enough to enable me to live a normal life, so I don't bother with daily medications for chronic pain. I usually only use compound pain cream locally to alleviate intense pain. For a few years, I walked with a cane much of the time, which helped to relieve some of the pressure on my right hip, but also helped me to avoid falling when I had symptoms of light-headedness, which happened several times a day. I was able to stop using the cane after finding the right physical therapy regimen to strengthen my hip, and finding the right medication to lessen my episodes of syncope. However, I have recently started using it again due to more frequent hip subluxations. I had found the right balance of weight and muscle tone, but am losing the muscle tone and weight due to problems with my digestive tract, so I am now having consequences of the low muscle tone.

I wear silver ring splints to keep my fingers from over-extending, dislocating, or subluxing (partial dislocation), but they are expensive and the weight loss has resulted in me losing several of them. I am unable to sit or stand for very long without needing to change position every few minutes. I am unable to do things overhead, and sometimes require assistance from my husband for basic care tasks. My son helps me to color my hair when necessary. I have constant unbearable neck pain, which makes reading, watching television, typing, and working on the computer painful.

In December of 2009, I made the decision that I simply could no longer work and continue to take care of my medical needs, so, I went out on long-term disability. I received a decision from the Hartford Group Insurance approving my disability without a long wait, but was initially denied social-security disability, and had to appeal for reconsideration. Thankfully, at my appeal hearing, the Judge approved my disability.

I was once very active, and went to the gym five days a week. I loved hiking, wildlife photography, and country dancing. I was reduced to having to use a cane and/or a wheelchair to get around, but slowly but surely I was getting my mobility back. I had started with physical therapy in a warm therapy pool, and then progressed to working out in my own pool, then working with a physical therapist and doing the recommended exercises at home, and lastly, I moved on to doing some Pilates and walking workouts at home. I am no longer doing these as I have been too sick and injury prone. I hope to get back in a warm water pool soon, and start over. When I was working out, I added in some strength training. As my muscles learned to take some of the pressure off of my joints, and my weight went down, I became more mobile, and that mobility was a blessing. Unfortunately, I have now lost too much weight due to severe gastric issues over the past year, and now I am beginning to lose the muscle tone that was helping to stabilize my joints.

I was never very heavy, but even an extra ten or fifteen pounds means a lot to fragile hypermobile joints. When I was healthier, I was down to 120 lbs., and on my 5'4" frame, that is the right amount of weight for me, so that I didn't overtax my joints. I knew that even with the increased mobility, and the weight loss, I could not and should not walk long periods at the mall or on the street, as those surfaces are too hard on fragile joints, but by staying mobile with workouts at home, and in the pool, I was able to regain some of my lost mobility at least temporarily. Unfortunately, with the increased weight loss from the digestion issues, I have a whole new set of issues as an "underweight" EDSer.

I use a wheelchair for longer walks outdoors or at malls or convention centers, and I am grateful for the freedom the chair provides. Without it, I would not be able to shop at the outlets or go to the board walk, so for me, the chair is its own form of freedom, but so is moving around on my own when I can.

I hope this narrative does not come across as complaining. Yes, living with Ehlers-Danlos Syndrome can be difficult and painful, but I try to look at it in as positive a light as possible. I have

EDS, but EDS does not have to have me. I wake up in the morning and force myself to decide whether I will stay in bed and cry about my condition, or get up and live my life to the fullest.

I am a born-again Christian and love the Lord with all my heart. I spend my days with God in prayer, bible reading, and whatever else He would have me to do. I am an amateur photographer, so I spend some time taking pictures. I enjoy bird watching and reading, so I do a good bit of both. I love writing, so I got voice software and committed myself to writing this book, in hopes that it would help others who had been newly diagnosed with this disease to find hope and understanding. I also raise awareness for Ehlers-Danlos Syndrome. These activities help to keep me from getting too caught up in myself and my medical problems.

Jeremy Thurman (Kyphoscoliosis Type)

Jeremy Thurman has Ehlers-Danlos
Syndrome Kyphoscoliosis Type (Formerly EDS
Type VI). Jeremy was 10 years old at the time of
my interview with his father, Joe Thurman. Many
of my readers may know Jeremy and Joe through
Facebook connections. Jeremy's dad has given me
permission to use his real name in this book in an
effort to raise awareness for EDS in general and his
son's battle with EDS in particular.

Jeremy was born without much muscle tone,
and with a curved back. The doctor ran her finger
down his spine, but didn't do any follow-up. His
father said he felt "like a little ball of mush" and
like "he had no bones." The doctors just ignored
the strange findings. At Jeremy's six week check-
up, they heard a clicking in his hip, so they
scheduled a follow-up visit, at which there was no
hip click.

Mentally, Jeremy was advanced. He used
his first computer at 8 month old, began reading at
one year old, and spoke clearly at two years old.

Eventually, after Jeremy broke his femur
twice at two years old, the doctors tested Jeremy for
all chromosomes. Around the same time,
Department of Children and Family Services
(DCFS) was called in, and they had to explain
Jeremy's injuries to them.

Jeremy used fixed ankle/foot orthotics
(AFO) and a new back brace, but a dip in the
ground caused his leg to break because he couldn't

move well with the orthotic. Joe fought for soft
AFOs, so that Jeremy could flex his foot up and
down, and they did finally agree to make one with a
hinge, so that Jeremy's ankle could flex. Since
then, his muscle tone has increased and he has
stopped falling. He was even able to run after they
changed it.

Jeremy was misdiagnosed with NM before
receiving his Ehlers-Danlos diagnosis. With NM,
surgical anesthesia is potentially deadly. Unusual
scarring was referred to a geneticist when Jeremy
was almost three years old. Maria C. Willing,
M.D., PhD. an expert in pediatric genetics and an
EDS specialist, diagnosed Jeremy with EDS Type
VI.

At the time of my interview with Joe,
Jeremy had already undergone approximately
thirteen surgeries. Eight of which were on his back.
He has the surgery every six months to adjust for
length, and he often gets released the same day and
returns to school within days. Jeremy refuses to
take pain meds for more than a day. Only when his
leg was broken did Jeremy use a wheelchair.

Jeremy has paper thin skin like tissue paper.
He does not bruise easily, but his skin breaks open
very easily. He busts his knees and elbows open
frequently, so Joe always has bandages and steri-
strips on hand. Jeremy has huge scars on his knees
and elbows, but the back scars from surgery are not
too bad.

Jeremy does have problems with
dislocations. When Joe holds his hand, he can feel

the bones pulling apart in Jeremy's hand. Jeremy's arm popped out of the socket in bed, but he was able to reduce the dislocation himself. Joe said it popped so loudly, that it woke him up. His fingers are also hypermobile.

Jeremy has always had a positive attitude and outlook about his health difficulties. However, EDS makes him look at life differently. On his seventh birthday, he said he wanted to be normal and not have to wear a brace. As he gets older, he worries more. Jeremy is a bright child, who stays on honor roll. He plays video games, reads, sings, and plays harmonica. He is a child who just happens to struggle with a very serious genetic disorder.

Leigh Barnett[1] (Hypermobility Type)

Leigh Barnett has Ehlers-Danlos Syndrome Hypermobility Type. Below is her story in her own words. She went from the care of an over-protective mother, to that of a loving husband, who encouraged her to begin to live her life more fully, but it took a life altering accident to really remind her how precious life is.

Leigh:
When I was diagnosed, I asked my mom if I could still have my dream, to be an astronaut. She laughed and told me "You better pick something else." This is when my mom went overboard with this idea of "protecting the joints" by putting me in a wheelchair, when I didn't need it. She just felt that walking would mean my joints might dislocate and if I used a wheelchair, I would prevent that. She even went so far as to get the State of Texas to pay to convert a van for me so that I could turn the vehicle on with a button, change gears with a button, put the parking brake on with a button, and drive with my hands. It was just over the top. As a result, I was coddled and made to feel afraid for my joints.

I was made to lead this sheltered life; my favorite thing, roller coasters - would be something I would never be allowed to experience anymore. I spiraled into depression, and gave myself pity parties daily. When I met my husband however, he encouraged me to stop using the wheelchair and it was probably the best thing I ever did for myself.

---
[1] Name has been changed to protect identity.

Still, back around 2000, I was living with my new husband and still was throwing daily pity parties and feeling sorry for myself for having EDS. I was treating it as if it was a curse. I was out of the wheelchair, but still using the handicapped equipped van. Things all changed when I was coming home from having lunch with my husband where he worked. I remember looking at the light ahead and it was green. It was then that I was cut off by an impatient driver and after evading an accident, I accelerated back to continue through the green light - except now it was red. I blew through the busy intersection going about 35-40 mph. I bounced off six cars and totaled my handicap van, which had been re-built like a tank. I should have broken every bone in my body, I should have died. However, I also discovered something about my EDS, my joints will dislocate before the bone will break. Nevertheless, I walked away, well more like limped away from an accident that should have taken my life.

It was then that I saw the bright side of having EDS....and it changed my entire outlook on EDS, life, everything. I made a symbolic "pact" with my EDS. I decided that if it keeps doing what it did during the accident, I will never complain about it again. My EDS has held up its end of the bargain, and I've held up mine. I'm at peace with my EDS. I still struggle with the years I spent in a wheelchair, I have to rebuild my muscles, get muscle tone, or face having many of my joints replaced. It's motivated me like nothing else, but I've learned over the years that I can do anything.

I hear people say that they wish they didn't have EDS, that it's a curse, that you would do anything to not have it; I used to feel like that in fact, but I feel differently now. If I didn't have EDS, I wouldn't be the person I am today. EDS makes me feel unique in a world where everyone tries to be "normal", like "everyone else." I like being unique. Oh, and roller coasters? They are totally not "off limits" like my mother made me believe. I make sure to ride them in fact, I may pay for it later, but life is a roller coaster, and if I choose to not ride them, I would be denying myself from living - a denial that I would regret for the rest of my life. We only live once and it's short - enjoy it. I'll happily trade a little pain for the rush and excitement that it brings, after all - that's life. I'll be darned if I'm going to live my life on the sidelines like I used to, after all, that got me in the position I'm in now. I spent half my life on the sidelines, it stinks. While everyone tried to convince me otherwise, I discovered that having EDS is not a reason to just give up.

Leigh has learned some very important lessons about life from her EDS. She learned not to quit, she learned to seek out the good in things, and even to take risks. I certainly wouldn't recommend that all EDSers go out and ride roller-coasters, especially not those of us with serious spinal issues like Chiari malformation or basilar invaginations, but it certainly cannot hurt for us to look for ways to enjoy our lives and live them to the fullest, even if we are confined to a wheelchair or have to use a walker. We must live our lives, not just go through the motions.

Dana James[2] (Kyphoscoliosis Type)

Dana James has Ehlers-Danlos Syndrome Kyphoscoliosis Type (Formerly EDS Type VIA). Below is her story in her own words. She has suffered with severe medical issues throughout her life, but is determined to make the most of her life, and to fight for her life even when the odds seem stacked against her.

Dana:

My symptoms started at birth. I was born a floppy baby with both hips dislocated, hip dysplasia, scoliosis, and severe hypotonia (I was resuscitated and was given an adrenalin injection straight to the heart). They thought I was autistic which made some sense, because autistic babies often have low muscle tone. It turned out that I had Asperger's syndrome, in addition to EDS - but didn't learn of it until adulthood.

They put me into Bock's aparat. I started walking late because of it.
My earliest memory is of the pain. I had pain all over but mostly in my joints and spine. I always thought everyone had it and that there was something wrong with me, because I couldn't cope with the pain like everyone else could. Nobody ever told me that it was not normal. I had subluxations and dislocations. It started with the right hip and I never told anyone, because I thought it was normal and everyone dealt with the same things.

---

[2] Name has been changed to protect identity.

31

The doctors only provided medical care for the scoliosis. They blamed it for every single symptom I suffered. When I was 13 they tried to straighten it and something went wrong at the C5-C6 level. I became a vegetable, dependent on a respiratory machine. They were sure I was going to die, but I survived.

After that, I became a part-time wheelchair user. Of course, I had all the symptoms of EDS III, but it is often considered to be the mildest form of EDS, and the doctors always claimed it was just neurosis. When I was fainting because of the pain, every single day on the school bus, they said it was just school anxiety, so they did nothing for me. I was not allowed at physical education lessons at school but had physiotherapy for the spine. I didn't know then that I was dealing with worsening EDS symptoms.

I was a pianist and they called me a wunderkind. Music was my life, I couldn't imagine I could do anything else. But in my late teens (about 16) I had to give up due to pain, finger dislocations, and other issues. I started to take morphine for the pain, which I took for 10 years. I couldn't take it anymore after I had my gallbladder removed because morphine causes bile duct crumps which causes pancreatitis, which I now know leads to death in Kyphoscoliosis type.

Many times I was close to death. Breathing failures, heart failures, bile duct dysfunctions - every diarrhea was and is life threatening to me. They used to say it's all because of spinal cord damages caused when I was 13.

I have mitral, aortal, and tricuspid valve prolapse, heart aneurysm, left heart fibrosis, tachycardia, and artial fibrillation. I also have high blood pressure. Further tests showed constant anemia, low resistance to infections (used to get interferon and immunoglobulin thru IV), urinary incontinence, organ prolapse, dysautonomia, severe hypotonia, enteritis, gastrointestinal hemorrhage, polyps and many other medical issues, the rest of which are not too bad. Of course my joints are in a horrible state, but you cannot die from that.

And of course I've always had physiological depression because of lysyl hydroxylase deficiency and serotonin effect. I cannot eat normal food, I depend mostly on special fiber feedings. I have uterus mucosa cancer caused by EDS and take chemo.

I wasn't diagnosed with EDS until age 36. I was diagnosed by a rheumatologist at the national Institute of Rheumatology in Warsaw. I was diagnosed with a combination of Brighton and Beighton scale, clinical tests and skin biopsy. I learned that I was the first EDS Type VIA (Kyphoscoliosis Type) diagnosed at the Institute of Rheumatology, actually I was the first EDSer diagnosed there.

I didn't have to learn to accept EDS, as I never knew any other life. I was born with it, so EDS was always there. I always thought I could live despite it but now it's just a fight for life and death. I'm winning so far.

Stephanie Jones[3] (Hypermobility Type)

Stephanie Jones has Ehlers-Danlos
Syndrome Hypermobility Type (Formerly EDS
Type III). Below is her story in her own words.

Stephanie:

My family always laughed about the odd
quirks which seemed to follow us around: the
clumsiness, the growing pains, the party tricks.
Nothing ever seemed worth looking into, not when
there were so many other health concerns floating
around the family tree. At least, not at first.

I always knew there was something different
about me in comparison to the kids I grew up with.
Memories of being too tired to play in kindergarten
from joints that wouldn't cooperate, constant
migraines, and a body that felt like it was controlled
by someone else just didn't seem to be concerns my
classmates faced. However, the general consensus
alternated between "it's all in your head" and
"that's just how our family is." So, my family and I
persevered. Looking back EDS was affecting my
life as a child but by no means controlling it. I
made friends, did well in school, and thirsted after
whatever knowledge I could get my hands on. If I
wasn't doing my chores, odds are you'd find me
lost in a book, a journal, or a daydream.

It wasn't until my high school years that my
condition began to grow more severe. Suddenly,
things like getting out of bed and holding a pencil
seemed like insurmountable tasks as my joints

---

[3] Name has been changed to protect identity.

34

deteriorated. Thus began my battle. My friends from elementary school weren't sure how to make the adjustment from my elementary school health to my high school struggles. Add to that a switch from the public school system to home schooling and, one by one, I watched my social network disappear.

Getting diagnosed with anything is a challenge in my hometown. The doctors care, but there are too few of them and too many patients to spend enough time learning about rare conditions when the everyday conditions already have them swamped. We tested vitamin levels, suggested weight loss, explored the possibility of depression. The only success we made, though, was my developing a wariness and distrust of the medical profession.

As a young girl, I couldn't understand why no one could make it better. How could anyone assume this was the life, filled with its pain, frustration, and illness, which I would actively want? I felt betrayed and it began to show.

I wish I could say I handled it with grace. I didn't. To add to the multitude of symptoms my EDS was adding to my life, I began a slippery slope into my own battle with depression as the doctors became more and more mystified. After years of being told that it was all in my head, add to that the stress of teenage life and family, so I reached out for any life preserver I could find. In my case, with the isolation my health had brought me, I found self-injury. High school and freshmen year of college was a blur of assignments, illness, and harm as I fought to make sense of my life amidst a world with no answers, until my first summer home from college arrived. Prior to making the 2,000 mile trek to college, my family doctor, shaking his head at my medical questions that still remained unanswered put in a referral for a geneticist, to be seen as soon as I returned home from school.

With much apprehension my mom took me down to Toronto to meet Dr. V. I walked in and met her and her intern (fresh from school I was the first patient he sat in on) and as we sat talking Dr. V smiled. At the end of our appointment I had a name – Ehlers-Danlos Syndrome. I had actually suspected it for a while but to have a name was so freeing and Dr. V agreed. Not that a diagnosis made everything better, I still had MRI's, ECG's, PT, and a variety of other letters now entering my life. The potential for chronic, recurring health problems for the rest of my life (currently fighting for POTS and Raynaud diagnosis), as well as the reality that, just like I had been saying all along, there was no magic pill to cure me.

Yet, at the same time, everything changed with that diagnosis. Being able to find out what was in my head and what wasn't, gave me the courage, along with the encouragement of my new and amazingly accepting friends to get the help I needed and get healthier mentally. I've now been free from self-injury for almost a year.

I've also found the strength to look for the things EDS has given me. Looking back it was far too easy to see what chronic illness takes: energy, health, friendship, driving, etc. On a bad day, the list could be a mile long. However, I'd be lying to say I've never received anything good from EDS as well, not saying I don't often imagine life without the limitations of this condition but since it's here I may as well find the blessings.

Because EDS has introduced me to a whole new community of people whose awesomeness I can't even begin to describe. Both in the online world of zebra's who jump in and support one another and in real life with the people, I am embarrassed to admit, I would have been too busy to notice if my body hadn't forced me to slow down.

EDS has also taught me to be more patient, more empathetic, and to have a better sense of humor. I mean, after all, some days with EDS all you can do is laugh (and pray the ribs stay in place). Even better, learning these lessons has shown me my passion for helping those who live on the fringe. As a result, I'm in school going for my M.A. in counselling.

Finally, EDS has taught me that it's okay to wait. I've tried going with the first doctor and been ignored for years. I tried to make it work with a guy only for him to say he couldn't handle someone who is chronically ill. However, I've found a doctor who listens and this summer I'm going to be married to the love of my life, whose biggest concern about my illness is how he can help me the most, while keeping me independent.

Life is truly what you make of it. Some people go through life never knowing the cards they were dealt, some of us get a sneak peak and find things like EDS in our hand. In the end though, it's not what cards you've been given but how you play them and finding ways to enjoy the ride.

Part III

Coping

When dealing with a disabling chronic condition, you will receive many different suggestions for ways to cope and improve your life. No two people will respond in the same way to any of those suggestions. However, I have found one thing that seems to be almost universally helpful, and that is to be present in the moment. Pain can easily become overwhelming when we think of it as something that will never go away, but when we break it down into smaller increments, we are able to handle it. There is a cliché used in Alcoholics Anonymous "one day at a time," and sometimes they will break it down to one hour at a time, or even one minute at a time. We can handle almost anything for one minute, so when the pain gets overwhelming, think in minutes not years.

Jesus tells us "Take therefore no thought for the morrow: for the morrow shall take thought for the things of itself. Sufficient unto the day is the evil thereof." (Matthew 6:34 KJV). Everyone knows that we cannot change the past, and the future is not yet here, so it is best to concentrate on the here and now. Unfortunately, though, there are times when we cannot seem to shut our minds off, so we relive past event in our heads, or we obsess about the future, and what we want for ourselves or for our children. When this happens, after much practice, I am now able to refocus on what I can do today to work towards my goals. I do not strive for perfection, I simply do the best I can to live for today.

There are many other ways of coping with a chronic illness, not the least of which, include finding ways of relieving stress. As previously discussed, focusing on the present will relieve some stress. Another way to deal with stress is physical exercise. Although exercise may be difficult for EDSers, it is beneficial to find a method of exercise to help you improve your physical and mental outlook. Exercise in a warm water therapy pool is ideal if you have access to one, but other forms of light cardio, strength training (with light-weights), and Pilates can be beneficial.

Finding a good support system is important. Sometimes, family members and former friends are not as supportive as we think they should be. When we don't get the support we need from those closest to us, we can turn to support groups. Those groups can include people you meet online or in person. Facebook provides those support groups for many EDSers, there are quite a few groups on Facebook where EDSers can talk about the issues that are affecting them. Many of those groups are listed in the Appendix of this book which includes the internet addresses. Butyoudontlooksick.com is another online resource for people suffering with chronic invisible illnesses, and they have many EDSers in their support network. Some EDSers write blogs, and that not only helps them by enabling them to share what is bothering them, it also helps their readers to feel less alone. The Ehlers-Danlos National Foundation lists some local groups where EDSers can meet in person. I have never been to one of those groups, because, unfortunately, there are none in my area. I was, however, able to go to one of the Ehlers-Danlos

National Foundation conferences, which was a great experience and introduced me to many new friends, and allowed me to meet face to face with old friends from Facebook who understand my daily struggles.

Progressive relaxation is an effective means of reducing stress and promoting sleep. I use progressive relaxation to help me get to sleep. I still use medication for sleep on occasion, but I find that most nights I am able to combat my insomnia by concentrating on relaxing each body part, starting with my toes and working my way up. I have been using progressive relaxation since I was a teenager.

Spirituality and prayer can also help us through hard times. The church can offer a sense of community where you can find understanding, and even learn to forgive yourself for being less-than-perfect. "He will regard the prayer of the destitute, and not despise their prayer." (Psalms 102:17 KJV). I am not suggesting that by prayer all your physical ailments will be healed, but I am suggesting that if you lean on the Lord, you are never alone in your struggle.

Godly meditation is another option and can be used in conjunction with prayer or alone. Many studies have shown that meditation provides many health benefits, including reducing stress. "I will meditate also of all thy work, and talk of thy doings." (Psalms 77:12 KJV).

When dealing with something as complicated and multifaceted as Ehlers-Danlos syndrome, it takes many different methods to help us cope. So, I suggest trying anything you think might work, and then continuing with the ones that work best for you.

Once I learned to accept that I have Ehlers-Danlos syndrome, I was able to come to terms with it. That acceptance was necessary for me to move on with my life, and stop obsessing over my EDS. It was easy to get caught up spending every moment researching EDS and the effects it was having on me, but in doing that, I was neglecting the rest of my life. Now EDS is something I have, but I do not let it have control over my life. It would be easy to spend every day on the internet talking to my EDS friends, doing research and obsessing over what might happen to me, but I have learned to compartmentalize it. I give myself time for EDS research and for commiserating, but I limit that time, so that it does not take over my life. I make time for God, family, and friends. They keep me sane.

1 Solis, MS., Java O. "Ehlers-Danlos Syndrome." My UHC. UnitedHealthcare, 2006. Web. 05 Jan. 2010. <https://healthatoz.myuhc.com/portal/Atoz/common/standard/transform .jsp?requestURI=/portal/Atoz/ency/ehlers-danlos_syndrome.jsp>.
2 Ehlers-Danlos National Foundation Staff. "What Are the Types of EDS?" Ehlers-Danlos National Foundation. Ehlers-Danlos National Foundation Staff. Web. 12 Jan. 2011. <http://www.ednf.org/index.php?option=com_content&task=view&id=1 348&Itemid=88888969>.
3 Tinkle BT, Bird HA, Grahame R, Lavallee M, Levy HP, Sillence D. 2009. The lack of clinical distinction between the hypermobility type of Ehlers–Danlos syndrome and the joint hypermobility syndrome (a.k.a. hypermobility syndrome). Am J Med Genet Part A 149A:2368–2370.
4 Ehlers-Danlos National Foundation. Ehlers-Danlos Medical Resource Guide. Ehlers-Danlos National Foundation, 2010. Print.
5 Staff, Mayo Clinic. "Ehlers-Danlos Syndrome: Complications - MayoClinic.com." Mayo Clinic. 20 Apr. 2010. Web. 12 Jan. 2011. <http://www.mayoclinic.com/health/ehlers-danlos-syndrome/DS00706/DSECTION=complications>.
6 Staff, Mayo Clinic. "Ehlers-Danlos Syndrome: Causes - MayoClinic.com." Mayo Clinic. 20 Apr. 2010. Web. 12 Jan. 2011.

<http://www.mayoclinic.com/health/ehlers-danlos-syndrome/DS00706/DSECTION=causes>.
7 Arthritis Foundation. Fibromyalgia. Ehlers-Danlos National Foundation, 2008. Print.
8 Létourneau, DMD, Yves, Pérusse, DMD, MD, Rénald, and Buithieu, DMD, MSD, Hélène. Oral Manifestations of Ehlers-Danlos Syndrome Abstract <http://www.cda-adc.ca/jcda/vol-67/issue-6/330.html>
9 Selina McKee. "US patients: seven-year wait for rare disease diagnosis." Pharma Times Online. 10 Apr. 2013. Web. 12 Jan. 2011. <http://www.pharmatimes.com/Article/13-04-10/US_patients_seven-year_wait_for_rare_disease_diagnosis.aspx>.

Appendix

Helpful Resources and Internet Links

This is a link to Dr. Brad Tinkle's latest book about EDS and Hypermobility Syndrome:

> http://www.amazon.com/Hypermobility-
> handbook--Management-Ehlers-Danlos-
> syndrome/dp/098257715X/ref=sr_1_2?s=bo
> oks&ie=UTF8&qid=1329141732&sr=1-2

These organizations, offer information about EDS:

Ehlers-Danlos National Foundation
  http://www.ednf.org/
EDS Network CARES Foundation
  http://ww.ehlersdanlosnetwork.org/
These are some Facebook groups devoted to EDS:
EDS fight for a cure
  http://www.facebook.com/groups/edsfightfo
  racure/
EDS friends
  http://www.facebook.com/groups/12883232
  7171082/
EDS Moan and Groan Clubhouse
  http://www.facebook.com/groups/28305956
  8428681/
EDS Neck Surgery Group
  http://www.facebook.com/groups/16440683
  3583472/
EDS Network
  C.A.R.E.S. http://www.facebook.com/#!/pag
  es/EDS-Network-CARES/295238396730
EDS Today (Ehlers Danlos Syndrome)

http://www.facebook.com/#!/groups/EDStod
ay/

Ehlers Danlos - Ladies Only
http://www.facebook.com/groups/29045128
7649985/

Ehlers Danlos Awareness
http://www.facebook.com/#!/groups/358792
522065/

Ehlers Danlos Syndrome type
3 http://www.facebook.com/#!/pages/Ehlers
-Danlos-Sy
ndrome-type-3/126241787394071

Ehlers Danlos Syndrome
http://www.faceook.
/#!/groups/2210965239/

Ehlers-Danlos Support Group
http://www.facebook.com/#!/groups/152615
741473177

Ehlers-Danlos syndrome & hypermobility
syndrome looking for friends
http://www.facebook.com/groups/EDS.and.
HMS.looking.for.friends/

Ehlers-Danlos Syndrome--advice on the best way
we get our joints back
http://www.facebook.com/groups/11848524
4864819/

Loosely Speaking: Ehlers-Danlos Anthology
http://www.facebook.com/groups/looselyspe
aking/

Raising Children with EDS-Ehlers Danlos
Syndrome
http://www.facebook.com/groups/26431150
7194/

Support Ehlers Danlos Syndrome
http://www.facebook.com/#!/groups/323535
01203/

Zebras For Life
    http://www.facebook.com/groups/hearhoove
    sthinkofzebra.EDS/
Zebras Need Zebra
    http://www.facebook.com/#!/groups/158252
    460691/
Zebras R Us
    http://www.facebook.com/#!/groups/168190
    497410/

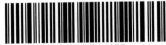

Made in the USA
Lexington, KY
05 February 2019